HOW TO WIN AT THE GYM

THE ESSENTIAL GUIDE FOR NEW GYM MEMBERS AND REFRESHER FOR OTHERS

Rudi Marashlian
and
Tracey Marashlian

Cover design by: Tracey Thatcher
Layout design by: Tracey Thatcher

Published by: Marashlian, Inc.

Visit the authors' website:

www.gofitnow.com

This book is dedicated to all health and fitness professionals who, on a daily basis, work to help people improve the quality of their lives through the use of natural remedies, nutrition and exercise.

ALSO BY RUDI MARASHLIAN

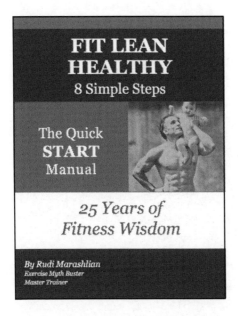

Fit Lean Healthy, 8 Simple Steps

- If you want to get leading-edge fitness knowledge that only personal training clients are usually fortunate enough to have access to...

- If you want to speed your progress through the roof...

Then this is the book for you.

Based on the same step-by-step method used on hundreds of personal training clients to get great results!

Visit **www.fitleanhealthy.com** to get this book!

TABLE OF CONTENTS

TABLE OF CONTENTS

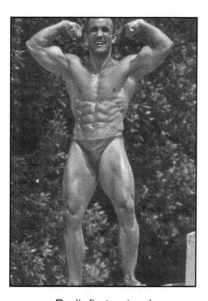

Rudi, first natural
bodybuilding show, 1992

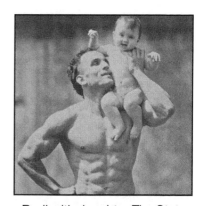

Rudi with daughter Tia. State
body building champ, 1993

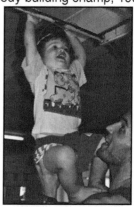

Rudi and son Obe, at
Mosman Gym 1993

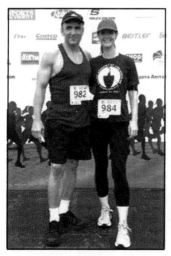

Rudi and Tracey at a
10K race, 2012

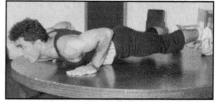

Rudi at Bodyline Gym,
Sydney in 1984

ABOUT THE AUTHORS

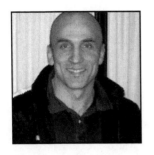 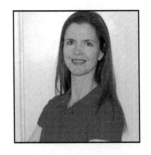

RUDI MARASHLIAN is an American College of Sports Medicine Health and Fitness Specialist and Exercise is Medicine practitioner. He is a graduate of the number one exercise science course of the University of New South Wales in Australia and has been training and coaching people professionally since the eighties.

Rudi's training philosophy is, "*The only real way to help anyone long term is to empower them through education, coaching and practice of correct and workable fitness basics. Train smart then train hard and use gradual steps to get there.*" He is the author of **Fit Lean Healthy, 8 Simple Steps**. You can contact Rudi via his website, **www.gofitnow.com**, he is happy to hear from anyone who wants to get more out of life through fitness.

TRACEY MARASHLIAN is an American College of Sports Medicine Certified Personal Trainer and has been involved in the fitness industry for over two decades. She writes leading-edge fitness articles professionally for local gyms and fitness blogs and runs a successful personal training business in Los Angeles with her business partner and husband, Rudi. She specializes in training women and helping them take charge of their bodies.

SUCCESS STORIES

"I thoroughly recommend Rudi as not only an excellent personal trainer, but he also merits even more praise as a training strategist specific to the needs of each individual."

Soren K

"I went from major back damage (slipped disk) to physically fit and comparable fitness-wise to my younger friends. In just a few months I was 'back to battery', beating my friends in punching contests, riding the hell out of a mechanical bull, and body surfing. Thanks Rudi.

Ryan D

"I bought *Fit Lean Healthy 8 Simple Steps*. I started reading and using it right away. The first thing that was a great win for me was to actually define my fitness goals. I had not done that at all before! With the goals in mind, then getting the mind-set of what it will take to achieve those goals, was so much easier. And doable. Even not having finished reading and using it, I have found myself so motivated, actually keeping in the discipline of the exercise time and already seeing results after just a couple of weeks,

Thank you so much, you guys did such a fantastic job on writing the book!!!"

Ximena S

SUCCESS STORIES

"When I started training, my overall goal was improved fitness, and yes, it's working! I'm dropping pounds and inches while toning muscle, gaining energy, stamina and smiles. My body is sculpting nicely, and my husband and friends are definitely noticing the changes. Many thanks Rudi!"

Sherryl B

"I love the scientific information regarding muscle groups and how to work on developing the underlying muscles which support the larger muscles. I feel I'm in safe hands with your guidance on the exercises, especially with emphasis on good form.

"So there is an overall improvement in weight, muscles, sleep and confidence. Feeling GREAT. Actually better than I have ever felt before. Not bad for fifty-five."

Robert S

"I feel like I have a lot more data than before about the exercises my body needs and how to use the gym properly to do those.

"I feel less intimidated and overwhelmed by the weight machines and vast array of exercises available to me!"

Triona M

INTRODUCTION

What are some of the very best tools we have at hand to create great health, improve appearance and remain youthful longer?

- A well-balanced exercise program designed specifically for you and done on a regular basis (by you)
- A personalized, well-balanced nutrition program that you actually follow
- Adequate sleep and rest

Fit, healthy people handle life very differently to those who are unfit. They have more energy and a positive outlook on life. If they experience an injury, set back, accident or illness because of bad luck or a momentary drop in the immune system they nearly always recover faster then their inactive, unhealthy counter-parts.

Once again, the 1-2-3 basic and natural formula for good health, fitness, anti-aging and longevity is:

- Regular balanced physical exercise
- Some good basic natural nutrition
- Adequate sleep and rest

The purpose of this book is to give you some important information on the first two tools - exercise and nutrition - to help make your gym-going experience successful and rewarding

Rudi Marashlian
Exercise Science, Applied Science
American College Sports Medicine Certified Health and Fitness Specialist

YOU JOINED THE GYM... NOW WHAT?

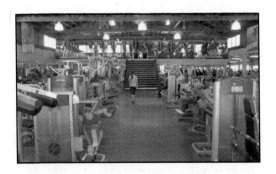

Congratulations, you joined the gym. This is a great step toward achieving your health and fitness goals.

Joining a gym doesn't automatically make you fit, strong or better-looking. It's what you *do* in the gym that counts - not what you wear or how much you paid to join or even that you arrive each day.

Gym membership these days are very inexpensive and because of this, they cannot include certain services you might need.

Gym membership usually includes:
- The right to visit and use the facility when the gym is open
- Access to the strength and cardio machines and any available group classes

Gym membership does not usually include:
- Instruction on how to use the equipment correctly
- A program based on your goals, strengths and weaknesses
- Diet help
- A fitness assessment
- Personal training

So what should you do now, especially if you are clueless about how to use the equipment or what activities to do so you can achieve your goals?

YOU JOINED THE GYM - NOW WHAT?

The four steps below have been put together to answer those questions for the new gym member who doesn't know where to start or what to do. It is an industry fact that leaving out any of these steps causes people to drop out early or fail at getting results.

Follow these next four steps in sequence to give yourself the best possible chance of getting great results.

THE FOUR STEPS TO SUCCESS

STEP #1 - Get the right information
Ideally you would read this book all the way through to get as much information as possible to help you get started the right way. Putting this information to use will help you get where you want to go.

STEP #2 - Manage your time, workouts and nutrition
Get organized and manage your time. Schedule and prepare your meals and workout times just as you would your business appointments. Your workouts will enhance all areas of your life, so make sure you grant them the importance they deserve.

STEP #3 - Focus on your goals
Be hard-working, focused and persistent towards what you are seeking to achieve in order to be successful. *Self-discipline* can be defined as being able to motivate yourself despite any negative emotional state or incoming obstacles. You are embarking on a big adventure, there will be difficulties along the way but the rewards are worth everything you have to go through. You won't make it unless you focus and stay focused.

STEP #4 - Take massive action now towards your goals
By *now* I mean the first four to eight weeks, which are crucial to setting up new habits regarding your workouts and the way you eat.

PART ONE - IMPORTANT FITNESS BASICS

THE RIGHT PLACE TO START - GOALS

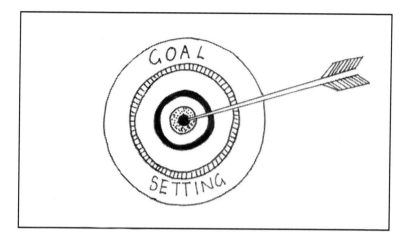

Goals are the driving, self-motivating forces that keep you going.

The first thing you should do is take a good look at why you joined the gym. What problem are you trying to solve?

Perhaps you want to look better to find a partner to share your life with. Maybe you want to improve your health to live a longer, happier and more youthful life. You might want to build big muscles so girls admire you and you never get sand kicked in your face at the beach!

Set realistic, attainable goals. Work out what you'd like to achieve and write your goals down on a piece of paper then post them somewhere you will see each day - like on the refrigerator.

GOAL ONE (set realistic goals for the first three months)

GOAL TWO (set realistic goals for the first six months)

GOAL THREE (set realistic goals for the first twelve months)

THE RIGHT PLACE TO START - GOALS

Keep in mind that within the first three months you will **FEEL better**, from three to six months you will start to **LOOK better** and see results, and from six to eighteen months you will **ACHIEVE your big goals**.

For right now, focus on the goal you set for the first three months. This is your most important goal and keeping it in mind will help you overcome the obstacles that fall in your path, especially as you start working out at the gym.

HOW TO OVERCOME THE URGE TO QUIT

If you ever lose hope or feel like dropping out, just remind yourself of why you started this journey - what did you really want to achieve?

If you are not getting the results you want or have hit a plateau, go back to *The Four Steps to Success* and see if one or more is either missing or not being applied.

SET REAL AND ATTAINABLE GOALS
HOW TO AVOID BECOMING DISCOURAGED

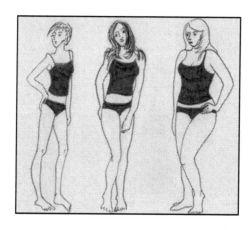

Ladies, don't get sucked in by magazines, infomercials or television ads and think you should look like the models they have posing in them. Some are genetically gifted, most are unrealistically photo-shopped.

Men should also follow this advice and avoid trying to look like the guys in muscle magazines who are often using performance-enhancing substances to create their huge physiques.

Set realistic goals for your age, health, genetic potential and living standards. If you do set the goal to be like a bikini model or professional bodybuilder but don't have the genetics (body type), willpower, time, money or desire to do whatever it takes to get there, then you will not attain that unrealistic goal.

Be happy with your strength, flexibility, cardio and improved quality of living. We don't all have the same genetics and appearance. Some people are small-boned and light naturally, others are heavier and more muscled. Everyone can improve their appearance and fitness levels to attain *their* best body. There are advantages to every body type, whether small, medium or large.

WHAT'S IN YOUR FITNESS TOOLBOX?

There are four basic **fitness tools** that can be used to achieve different health, fitness, rehabilitation, and sports results.

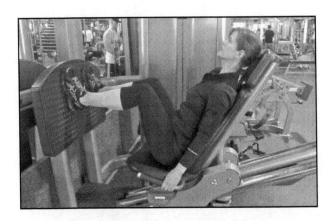

TOOL #1: STRENGTH TRAINING:

Strength training will help you look and feel good. It will also help you move and function well with strong and conditioned muscles.

Benefits of strength training - Muscle strength and tone: this affects how well you do the activities of daily living, your quality of life and your general appearance. The more conditioned your muscles are, the more calories you will burn. The stronger you become, the easier daily activities become and the less likely it will be to injure your back, knees and other vital areas of your body.

Examples of strength training activities:
- Body weight exercises, like push-ups
- Free weights exercises using bars and dumbbells, like a bench press
- Strength machines, like the leg press

WHAT'S IN YOUR FITNESS TOOLBOX?

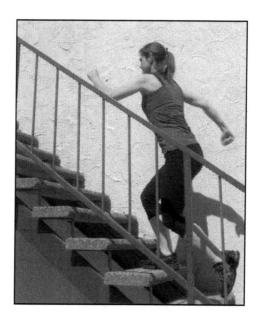

TOOL #2: AEROBIC/CARDIO TRAINING:

Aerobic or cardio training will help you feel good and improve your heart and lung conditioning.

Benefits of aerobic or cardio training - A healthier heart and lungs. The more heart and lung fitness and conditioning you have, the easier endurance activities like running, swimming and cycling will become. Cardio fitness helps increase your energy levels, and helps your heart, lungs, as well as blood and lymph circulation. Aerobic exercise also helps to burn calories.

Examples of cardio or aerobic training activities:
• Outside the gym - jogging, swimming, cycling, rowing, playing sports like soccer and basketball
• In the gym - treadmill, rower, bike, stair climber, elliptical, hand crank

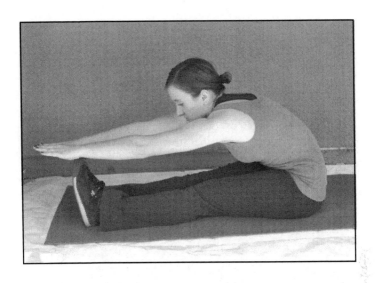

TOOL #3: FLEXIBILITY TRAINING:

Flexibility training (stretching) will help you move with ease. It improves your range of motion.

Benefits of flexibility training - Improved range of joint movement. The more flexible your joints and muscles are, the easier your daily activities become and the less likely it will be to injure your back, knees, shoulders and other areas of your body.

Examples of flexibility training activities:
• Yoga
• Pilates
• Scientific stretching exercises

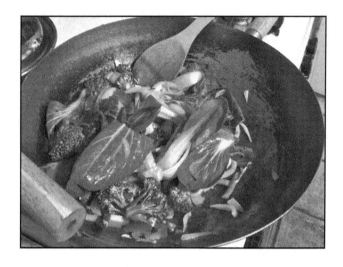

TOOL #4: NUTRITION - FOOD CONTROL:

Look, feel and function your best with purposeful eating.

Benefits of food control - Improved body composition, increased energy, better health. Hippocrates (Ancient Greek physician born 460B.C.) knew the effectiveness of food as a powerful healing tool. Food is not only a natural and powerful medicine but also a tool that can help create different conditions in the human body. Food can be used to aid exercise and sports performance, including recovery from illness and exercise or sports as well as being a key ingredient in fat loss, muscle building and increasing energy. If food is abused or misused it can lead to poor health, malnutrition, illness, heart disease, diabetes and obesity, to mention a few unhealthy conditions.

THE FITNESS TRIANGLE - A BALANCED PROGRAM

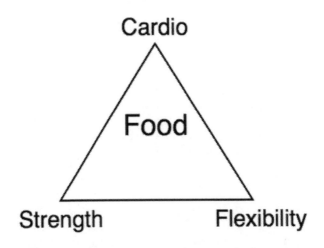

Make sure your fitness program is balanced. This would include using all four parts of the **FITNESS TRIANGLE.**

Each corner gives you a different result. How much of each you do or specialize in will affect the kind of results you get.

Your goals will determine which of the corners you will put more effort into, but all four will need to be covered in varying amounts.

For example, if you are training for a marathon you will focus mostly on cardio with some strength, flexibility and good nutrition. If you want to lose weight you'll need to mostly do strength and cardio with a bit of flexibility and also reduce the amount of food you eat. To body build your efforts will go into strength training and managing your food with some cardio and a little flexibility.

WHAT ACTIVITIES SHOULD YOU FOCUS ON?

Which fitness tools and how much of each will you need to do to achieve your goals?

If your goal is weight loss, should you be focusing on yoga (stretching)? If your goal is to tone up or build muscle, should you spend your workouts running on a treadmill (cardio)? The answer to these two questions is no.

Look over the goals in the following chart. Find the ones similar to yours then look across to find out which fitness tools you will need to focus on when you start working out.

	Tool 1	Tool 2	Tool 3	Tool 4
GOALS ↓	**STRENGTH TRAINING**	**CARDIO TRAINING**	**STRETCH TRAINING**	**NUTRITION**
Lose weight	Yes	Yes	No	Yes
Speed up metabolism	Yes	Yes	No	Yes
Build muscle	Yes	Some	Some	Yes
Tone muscles	Yes	Yes	Yes	Yes
Increase energy	Yes	Yes	Yes	Yes
Look good	Yes	Yes	No	Yes
Injury rehab	Yes	Yes	Yes	Yes
Improve health	Yes	Yes	Yes	Yes
Increase strength	Yes	Some	Yes	Yes

WEIGHT LOSS

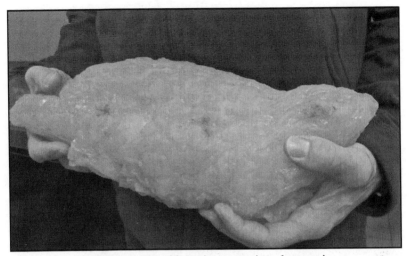

Five pounds of fat takes up a lot of space!

Weight loss is the main goal for a lot of people who join the gym. Technically, they want to reduce the amount of fat in their bodies and so decrease their size and improve their appearance.

To look good you will need to reduce fat and increase the amount of lean tissue (muscle) in your body. This will involve doing some strength and cardio training with changes to your diet. Muscle burns three to five times more calories than fat and that's why it's important to do strength training, especially for women.

EXERCISE IS MEDICINE
TREAT INJURY, DEPRESSION, DIABETES, HEART DISEASE AND MORE

Exercise is Medicine is an initiative launched by the American College of Sports Medicine and the American Medical Association that calls on physicians and other practitioners to prescribe exercise to their patients.

Research proves that exercise has a role in the treatment and prevention of more than 40 chronic diseases including diabetes, heart disease, depression, obesity and hypertension.

Exercise is Medicine is very strong in Australia where the national organization is working with doctors and nurses to make physical assessment a part of every patient visit.

The three guiding principles they follow are:

• Physical activity and exercise are important to health and the prevention and treatment of many chronic diseases
• Support the prescription of physical activity and exercise in health care settings
• Support the referral of patients to appropriately trained allied health professionals to deliver exercise treatment services

There is a growing number of personal trainers qualified to deliver the Exercise is Medicine program. The initiative is gaining popularity among the medical community with groups like Kaiser Permanente now recording information about patients' physical activity levels as a vital sign alongside blood pressure, pulse and temperature so they can be properly counseled by their doctors.

TONE AND STRENGTH

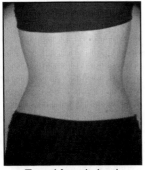
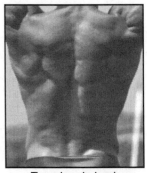

Toned female back   Toned male back

Toning is a gentle term which means to firm up muscles. The only way to do that is to challenge the muscles with some strength training, also known as resistance or weight training, or lifting.

Muscles are either growing (because of use, especially when you do resistance exercises) or shrinking (due to inactivity, aging or over doing the cardio - marathon running, for example, is known to strip muscle).

If you want to tone up, you essentially have to build muscle - increasing the amount of muscle mass of your body. Muscle is what shapes and firms the body. Without muscle, your body will be soft, saggy and unshapely (no matter how fat or "skinny" you may be).

Some advantages of toning up your body are:

- You will look firmer and tighter
- You will be stronger and better able to use your body in everyday situations like lifting loads, carrying children, pushing shopping carts, and so on
- You will increase your metabolism because muscle burns three to five times more calories than fat cells

BODY BUILDING

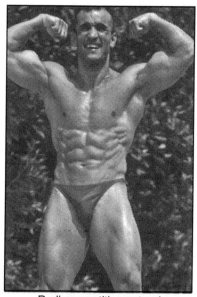

Rudi competitive natural
bodybuilder at 32

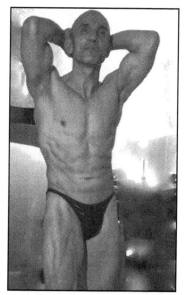

Rudi competitive natural
bodybuilder at 52

Anyone who is doing some sort of strength training or toning is really doing some form of body building to a degree, whether they know it or not. Muscles under load or stress increase in size (even if only slightly).

There are three types of body builders you will find in most gyms.

- The general population doing toning of strength exercise
- The recreational bodybuilder, mostly men trying to build medium to very large mass
- The competitive bodybuilder who is trying to build the largest mass possible with the lowest fat levels in order to win body building competitions

BODY BUILDING

The majority of gym-goers are doing some form of body building if they are trying to improve on strength and tone. The next large group are the recreational bodybuilders, mostly men trying to bulk up who can be seen to be taking extra protein and other supplements, but who do not enter bodybuilding competitions. Then we get the competitive bodybuilders who are the smallest group.

In the competitive bodybuilder category there are two types: the giant body builder people are used to seeing in muscle magazines (this person uses performance enhancing drugs to build giant muscles), and the natural bodybuilder (who uses natural supplements and will not have giant muscles, but more of a sports or athletic look).

Learning and understanding the basics of good form and technique is very important to ensuring you get optimum results with maximum safety

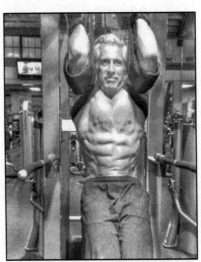

Our friend and successful natural body building champion, Tomas de la Milera. In his fifties and still looking great.

WOMEN AND WEIGHT TRAINING

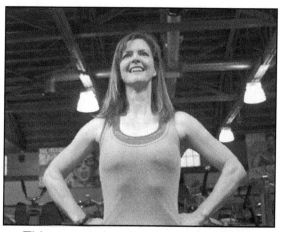

This woman has been weight training
hard for more than 20 years

Back in the eighties and nineties it was rare for women to do
strength training because of the false belief they had that
training with weights would cause them to bulk up and look
more like men than women.

We had many women come to our strength training gym in
Sydney looking to tone up, lose weight and look good because
all the aerobic activities and classes they did at other gyms
failed to deliver results. Luckily for them, we knew two things:

1. That **women don't bulk up** and get huge when they do
   strength training (unless they are using testosterone or other
   similar substance)

2. That **the only way women *can* tone up**, look great and
   improve their shape is to do some kind of strength training
   as part of their balanced program

WOMEN AND WEIGHT TRAINING

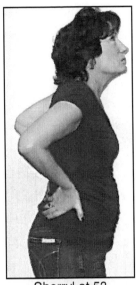

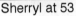
Sherryl at 53

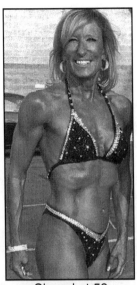
Sherryl at 58

It's never too late. Sherryl started weight training with us aged 57, applying the principles in this book. A year later she was winning trophies in figure competitions and looking better than ever before.

Today more women are aware of the benefits of strength training - increased bone density, better posture, tight muscles, a shapelier body, improved strength, among others - but there are still many who are afraid they will turn into a hulk if they start lifting weights.

Ladies, don't be afraid of the weights. Increasing the amount of muscle on your body will help you burn more calories every day and keep your fat levels down. It will give you a leaner, tighter physique, it will help you fit into smaller dress sizes and it will increase your confidence because you'll know you can rely on your body to do its job effectively in life.

ANTI-AGING FOR BABY BOOMERS

If you are 50 or older, is it too late to get into shape? Can you lose the flabby belly and improve your muscle tone? How about building muscle size and definition if you are a male?

The good news is *yes*, despite your age you can make very good changes and improvements to your health, fitness, appearance, energy and more, but it won't happen quite as fast as it may have happened when you were in your 20's.

Over the years we have helped many women in their 50's, and even older, who came to us with the problem of not being able to lose weight and wanting to improve appearance. Usually they'd tried everything that used to work in the past but found those things didn't work any more.

We've also seen many men in their mid-50's come in thinking it was too late or hopeless to try and build some muscle to look and feel better.

Getting the right information on diet and exercise and how to apply it well becomes more crucial as you age. How you apply it will depend on your age, genetics, injuries, and the type of goals you want to achieve. As your body changes, so too will your exercise program.

It's never too late to start working out. Anyone, even if they're over 50 can get very similar benefits to younger people, but they do need to progress more gently.

Three of the people featured in this book, including the author, are over 50 and they look great. Baby Boomers (those born between 1946 and 1964) don't want to be "old" and as more people over 50 start to exercise correctly and eat nutritious food, they are able to turn back their biological clocks and enjoy life like much younger people.

PART TWO - HOW TO GET STARTED
AND SURVIVE THE GYM

WHAT TO EXPECT WHEN YOU FIRST START WORKING OUT

The first 4 to 8 weeks are the most important with regard to your gym workout schedule. This is when you need to set up new habits like going regularly to the gym despite any and all urges or pulls from other areas of life. This is when you learn to be consistent and make going to the gym a priority in your life. People who don't do this, tend to drop out.

Keep in mind, you won't change your body completely in the first few weeks. It does take time. Most people will **FEEL** better within the first one to three months of regular training. They begin to **LOOK** better within the next three months, often they notice improvements earlier. The most important thing is that you don't give up and that you keep coming to the gym and exercising regularly no matter what.

If you challenge your body with exercise or activity it is very normal to experience some muscle soreness. This usually sets in within 24 to 48 hours. Stretching, movement, massage and light exercise all help to speed the recovery and healing process. Don't forget adequate protein in your diet can also help speed recovery.

Muscle soreness is not a good reason to avoid going to the gym. You can always exercise a different muscle group while the sore muscles recover.

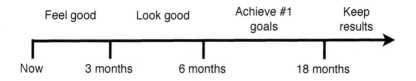

WHAT TO BRING TO THE GYM

WATER
It's a good idea to bring your own water especially if you are doing a lot of cardio or exercising during summer. Keeping your body hydrated will help it work better. If part of your goal is to lose weight or body fat then drinking enough water (about 8 to 12 glasses a day) is very important.

TOWEL
It's a good idea to bring a towel (a regular hand towel works well) to lay on top of gym equipment you are using. It not only keeps germs, sweat and body fluids off you but also helps to let others know that the space is in use if you walk away for a moment to get water or stretch.

VENTILATE - WEAR LIGHT CLOTHING
Would you drive a car with a blanket spread over the engine or radiator? Not likely, unless you want to overheat and possibly blow up your engine. The same applies to the human body when working out - less clothing is better when your body temperature rises.

As you get warmer in your workout, gradually layer off excess clothing like jackets, caps and hoodies so you can keep from overheating.

Some people have the idea that if you wear plastic around your abdomen or a plastic suite when you exercise you shed fat weight. This is completely false. It is a potentially dangerous practice and you will only lose water weight and most likely dehydrate. Fat loss happens with a combination of good diet and strength and cardio training done regularly.

WHAT TO BRING TO THE GYM

If the weather is cold outside layer clothes on as you cool down at the end of your workout to make sure you don't get too cold too fast.

SOME EXAMPLES OF GYM CLOTHING

Men:
Men typically wear shorts or track pants with sleeveless tops or T-shirts. Long track pants and long-sleeved shirts work well during the winter. Wear appropriate gym shoes.

If you like to run, get running shoes. Get cross trainers for gym classes and workouts or weight lifting shoes for those who just like to lift. Avoid wearing flip flops or open-toed shoes at the gym.

Women:
Women usually wear shorts, tank tops, T-shirts, capris, yoga pants, sweat pants and appropriate gym shoes. If you run, get running shoes. Get cross trainers for general gym classes and workouts. Try to avoid shorts that are very short or very baggy at the bottom of the legs (like basketball shorts) as you do sometimes put your body in positions that could cause embarrassment to you or others if your pants happen to be too revealing.

WORKOUT DIARY
A workout diary can be a very useful tool to motivate you and track your progress. You can record your body weight, girth, fat and strength measurements. For weight loss, fat loss or muscle gain it is also wise to log your food along with your workouts. You can use a standard exercise book or an app on your smartphone.

WHAT NOT TO BRING TO THE GYM

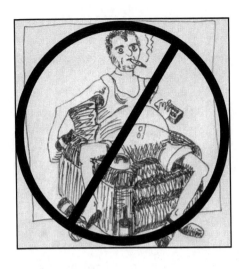

DIRT AND BODY ODOR
It's a good idea to wear some deodorant, use mouth wash or shower before mixing in with a crowd, especially if your work makes you dirty, sweaty or smelly and you come to the gym after work.

SMELLY GYM CLOTHES
Regularly change your workout clothes. Yes, we can smell you a mile away when you wear the gym clothes you sweated in two days ago. The accumulation of several days of dried up sweat and body odor is... (no swearing allowed).

STINKY ATTITUDE
This is your gym, your club, your space. You share it with others. Why spoil it for everyone by bringing your bad mood to your workout. It is easier and more fun to get along with others so if you are having a bad day, come to the gym (you'll always feel better after a workout) but leave the attitude at home.

WHAT NOT TO BRING TO THE GYM

THE WRONG CLOTHES CAN BE DANGEROUS
When you work out your body generates heat and needs to cool down to operate safely and effectively. Wearing too many clothes or the wrong type or some weird gimmick like plastic clothes, sauna suits or plastic around your waist to lose weight can only make you lose water, cause headaches, dehydrate you and possibly give you heat stroke, it will not result in fat loss!

Wear light clothing that breathes well and keeps you cool enough to avoid overheating.

DISTRACTIONS
Leave your iPad, magazines, novels, home work or anything else that can distract you from why you are really at the gym (to do a quality workout which will contribute towards you achieving your fitness goals). Do not waste your time. There are enough distractions at the gym with TV monitors and people to chat to without adding more for yourself.

HEAD PHONES
Doing workouts with head phones on is like driving with earplugs in - you need all of your senses when navigating and sharing the gym with others. Say someone calls out to warn you that you are about to hit your head on a bar or that your weight is about to fall off and strike someone working out near you, can you hear them? If you must have headphones on, turn the music down low enough so you can still hear others nearby.

GYM ETIQUETTE
HOW TO SURVIVE AT THE GYM

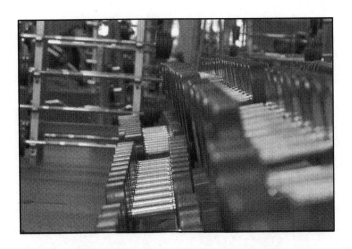

Pick up your weights. Would you believe there are some people in gyms who don't put their bars, weights and dumbbells away after they use them? They are usually the same characters who leave sweat puddles on bench seats or head rests and used paper towels on the gym floor. Don't be one of them.

It's not always true, but most offenders are usually new, inexperienced gym-goers. Gym pros and experienced gym-goers put their equipment back in the appropriate place when done and wipe down their bench after use, ready for the next person.

If you notice anyone chronically leaving their equipment out, let the gym manager know. Not only is it annoying, it's also a safety hazard when items are left about.

GYM ETIQUETTE
HOW TO SURVIVE AT THE GYM

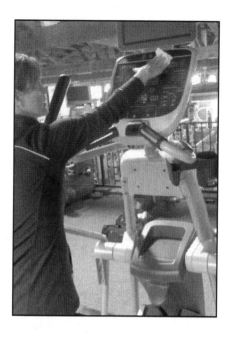

Clean off your sweat. This includes benches, strength and cardio machines, exercise mats, dumbbells and barbells. It is a good idea to wipe any sweat or potential germs off the bench, exercise mat or machine before and after you use it. Some people sweat a lot, some are sick or have a disease that they can pass on to you. Stay healthy and keep the equipment clean.

Always wash your hands thoroughly with soap and water before and after going to the bathroom and after your workout - this is not only good gym etiquette, but important for keeping you and others healthy at the gym.

GYM ETIQUETTE
HOW TO SURVIVE AT THE GYM

Sharing gym equipment. There will be times when you want to use a piece of equipment or machine but find that someone is using it or (possibly) resting, sleeping, texting, reading a book or anything else but working out on it. So what do you do?

Here's a simple format:

Ask politely if they are nearly finished with the equipment. Or, ask if you can work in with them (if you are doing the same exercise).

Most members will say yes. If it's a valid and fair no, it's usually because they are doing different exercises than you or they are using much heavier weights than you. If you asked politely and the person is outright rude, just let the gym manager know. It's rare but every gym has a jerk or two.

If you are the person using the equipment and someone asks to share, it's good gym etiquette to let another person work in with you. When you are done with a set and resting before the next one, instead of just sitting on the equipment, you can use the time to stretch out while the other person does a set. Not only is this better for you because you are getting more out of your gym time, it's also helpful to the other person.

Sometimes a personal trainer will be using the gym equipment with a client. The same rules apply - ask politely if you can work in with them and be willing to allow them to work in with you if asked (who knows, you might even learn something new to improve your own workout).

PART THREE - MAXIMIZE SAFETY
AND RESULTS

CHOOSING THE RIGHT TRAINER
ACCELERATE YOUR RESULTS

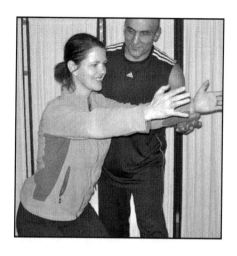

A very good trainer can set you up really well so you get maximum fitness results and safety in minimal time.

If you are not a fitness expert, how *can* you tell a great trainer from a bad or mediocre one? Here are some insider tips to help you.

Attributes of a Very Good Trainer

1. Ideally educated at university level in exercise science, sports science or kinesiology (the science of human movement)
2. Certified by one of the top three fitness certifying bodies - ACSM, NSCA, or NASM (these are the best out of over 300 certifying bodies in the United States)
3. Has insurance and an up-to-date CPR card
4. Has worked with people similar to you and can verify the results obtained (photos, testimonials)
5. Has a personality that you can easily get along with
6. Does continuing education with the top three certifying bodies (ACSM, NASM or NSCA)

7. Makes sure to educate you in the basics of fitness.
8. Does a thorough fitness assessment with you before training you, and works with your goals, strengths and weaknesses in mind
9. Keeps a training log to maximize your progress and safety

A bad trainer simply doesn't have the same attributes a good trainer has, but there are a few other tell-tale signs.

Additional Attributes of a Bad Trainer

Even one of these attributes is bad, but if you see a trainer with more, stay right away:

1. Has poor attention to exercise form (P.A.E.F.) and ends up giving bad advice, bad exercises and delivering zero results
2. Does not do a standard fitness assessment with new clients
3. Kills clients in the first session and gives advanced exercises to beginners (barbell squats or jumping up on boxes, for example). Clients can be seen vomiting or passing out during workouts
4. Spends session time talking about personal problems or a failing (or overactive) love life
5. Shows more interest in a cell phone, mirror, or in chatting with other gym members than in observing and helping the client

Do not hesitate to ask a potential trainer for proof of their education, certification, insurance and testimonials no matter who refers you to that trainer.

Bad personal trainers can be found anywhere, even in the most expensive gyms and if you don't know how to choose a good trainer, you could end up with a bad one. Bad training leads to poor results and, worse, possible injury.

THE RIGHT WAY TO DO A WORKOUT

It's essential to prepare the body before undertaking any vigorous exercise or activity. A simple way would be to do similar exercises or activities to those you will be doing in your workout but at a lower or lighter intensity or pace until your body temperature increases by about one to two degrees. This will better prepare your muscles and joints for more strenuous activities.

USE THE FIVE PARTS OF A WORKOUT IN SEQUENCE

PART ONE - DO WARM UP CARDIO: Do at least 5 to 10 minutes of any of these activities - brisk walking or light jogging, riding a stationary bicycle, using the elliptical machine or stepper, stepping up and down on small box until you break into a sweat and your body has warmed up.

PART TWO - DO WARM UP DYNAMIC STRETCHES: Do dynamic or moving stretches before you workout. Do 10 to 20 repetitions of each stretch. While standing, reach for the ground then stretch your arms above your head, for example. Maintain a steady motion and make sure you never bounce.

PART THREE - DO YOUR STRENGTH OR CARDIO WORKOUT: This is where you do the main part of your workout whether you are focusing on cardio or on strength or both.

PART FOUR - DO LIGHT CARDIO TO COOL DOWN: After you finish your workout do some easy, gentle cardio activity or exercises for 5 to 10 minutes, until your body starts to cool down and your heart rate reduces.

PART FIVE: DO STATIC STRETCHES: Lastly, do some static or hold stretches. Do each stretch 1 to 3 times. Hold each stretch for about 30 to 60 seconds. Hold at the point of slight discomfort.

THE RIGHT WAY TO DO A WORKOUT

SAFETY TIP: Only stretch the body *after* it has been warmed up. Cold muscles do not stretch as well and can pull if too tight or overstretched. Never bounce at the end of the stretch (called ballistic stretching) as this can strain muscles, create scar tissue and reduce flexibility.

USE THE FIVE PARTS OF A WORKOUT IN SEQUENCE

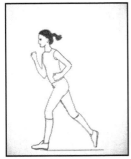

1. Cardio

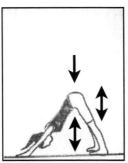

2. Dynamic Stretch

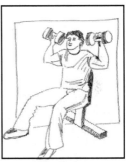

3. Workout

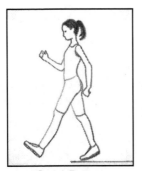

4. Cool Down

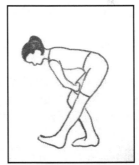

5. Static Stretch

HOW HARD SHOULD YOU WORK OUT?
LEVELS OF INTENSITY OR EFFORT

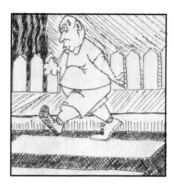

How do you monitor how hard or easy you need to exercise to keep it safe as well as effective?

Use a simple scale of exercise intensity. This scale applies to cardio, weight training or group classes.

Level 1 being super easy and **Level 10 being 100 percent hard** (this is where you can't do any more exercise with proper form).

If you only exercise at Level 1, you won't experience much change and will probably start to feel discouraged after a while.

Exercising at about a **Level 5 to Level 7 is a good way to start** if you are in good health, injury-free or have a doctor's approval to exercise.

Going at it to a Level 10 when you are new or have had a break might make you want to quit, and the whole point of exercise is to keep doing it to get results.

Stop if you feel dizzy, light-headed or nauseous until you are fully recovered. If you don't recover, seek medical attention as soon as possible.

MAXIMIZE RESULTS, MINIMIZE INJURY
THE FIVE GOLDEN RULES OF GOOD TRAINING

Rule 1 – BREATHE: Do not hold your breath during any type of exercise or movement. If you feel light-headed, dizzy or nauseous, stop the activity until fully recovered. Keep breathing.

Rule 2 – CORRECT FORM: Deliver perfect exercise form each and every time (once you learn it). Stop the exercise or activity any time your exercise form or posture cannot be maintained due to fatigue or for any other reason.

Rule 3 – EFFORT: Use the correct amount of force, effort or intensity to stay safe and get results.

- Work at 20 to 40 % of maximal effort if you are coming back from injury
- Work at 40 to 70% of maximal effort if you are injury-free and learning new exercises
- Work at 70% to about 90% of maximal effort if you are injury-free, highly conditioned and experienced with the exercise or activity
- Vary the exercise effort or intensity based on your age, physical condition, health, experience and goals

Rule 4 – PAIN: If at any time during exercise or activity you experience joint, muscle or nerve pain, stop immediately.

Rule 5 – REST: Rest fatigued muscles until they recover. This helps avoid over-training and gives the body enough time to heal and recover from tough training sessions.

CHECKPOINTS FOR CORRECT POSTURE

Checkpoint 1: FEET (applies to nearly all exercises)
- FRONT VIEW: Feet pointed straight ahead and shoulder to hip-width apart
- REAR VIEW: Feet flat on floor, pointed straight ahead

Checkpoint 2: KNEES (applies to nearly all standing exercises)
- FRONT VIEW: Knees pointed straight ahead, hip to shoulder-width apart
- SIDE VIEW: Knees slightly bent when standing. When squatting, knees kept behind toes
- REAR VIEW: Knees pointed straight ahead, not turned in or out

Checkpoint 3: LOWER BACK/PELVIS (applies to exercises that involve bending and squats)
- REAR VIEW: Top of both hips parallel to the ground, no tilt
- SIDE VIEW: Lower back in neutral position, spine slightly arched (natural curve)
- FRONT VIEW: Top of both hips parallel to the ground, no tilt

Checkpoint 4: SHOULDERS (applies to nearly all exercises)
- FRONT VIEW: Shoulders parallel to the ground, no tilt
- SIDE VIEW: Chest out, shoulders pulled back and down
- REAR VIEW: Shoulders parallel to the ground, no tilt

Checkpoint 5: NECK/HEAD (applies to exercises that involve bending and squatting)
- SIDE VIEW: Neck in neutral position, natural curve of the neck
- FRONT VIEW: Look straight ahead, no head rotation or tilt to the side
- REAR VIEW: Look straight ahead, no head rotation or tilt to the side

EXERCISE SAFETY - DO'S AND DON'TS

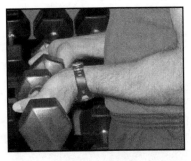 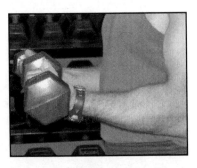

Do not over-extend a joint. To the left you see the wrists over-extending. To the right you see the correct way to hold dumbbells to avoid straining the wrists and elbows.

Do not over-bend (flex) a joint

Do not over-extend, over-straighten or lock a joint (hyperextension)

Do not bounce at the end of a stretch

Do warm up, stretch, workout, cool down and stretch with workouts (all five parts of a workout)

Do learn and apply perfect exercise form for each exercise

Do balance your workouts to include all three basic tools - strength, stretch and cardio exercises

Do breathe. Never hold your breath while exercising

Do challenge yourself gradually when you work out in order to improve and get fitter and stronger

FIVE FAMOUS FITNESS MYTHS

You can spot reduce a fat area like the abs

Are you trying to lose belly fat or trim your thighs? Doing 1000 sit-ups will *not* result in a six-pack or a skinny waist. Doing hundreds of squats alone will *not* give you slimmer thighs.

When you exercise you use your muscles, which sit *under* the fat layer you want to shrink. Reducing body fat is the answer to getting slim thighs and a smaller waist. This is done with strength and cardio exercises as well as diet.

Training with weights make women bulky

Only if they take muscle-building steroids along with eating excess calories. Lifting weights for women is the secret behind getting a great-shaped body and turning your body into a fat-burning machine 24/7. Do sets of 10 challenging reps to burn nearly twice the calories as using light weights.

You are too old to improve

If you are 50, 60 or even 70 or more years of age you *can* improve your health and fitness. It just takes a little longer and it won't be exactly the same or as easy as when you were 20.

All trainers are the same

Absolutely not! There are good, bad and "ugly" trainers. How can you tell? Go to page 32 "Choosing the Right Trainer". In Australia they have a grading system based on level of fitness education. Unfortunately, this does not exist in the USA and your average trainer is lightly educated.

Cardio is the best way to burn fat

Cardio is a great way to burn fat but you should also include weight training to build muscle. Muscle burns three times more calories than fat cells. Having more muscle means you burn more calories when you do cardio and it will turn your body into a 24/7 calorie-burning furnace. Diet is crucial to helping you burn fat, especially as you age.

PART FOUR - HOW TO USE THE GYM
EQUIPMENT AND WORK OUT

INTRODUCTION TO WORKOUTS

Of course, the reason you joined the gym was to have a place to work out so you could start achieving your health and fitness goals. Joining the gym and then not having a clue about what workouts to do defeats the purpose and usually results in an unused gym membership after a few weeks.

HOW OFTEN SHOULD YOU WORK OUT?

The American College of Sports Medicine (the ACSM sets standards for the fitness industry world-wide) recommends that adults should get at least **150 minutes** of moderate-intensity cardio exercise per week, they should do resistance exercise, functional fitness training and flexibility (stretching) **two or three days a week**.

How can you apply this information?

Follow the format for a complete workout (see **page 34** - *The Right Way to Do a Workout*) two, three or more times a week. If you are really trying to change your body you will need to work out at least three times a week, preferably more.

Here is a simple grid with two ways you could schedule your workouts to get the best results:

Workout Type	Weekly Schedule
Cardio only day Strength only day	Alternate days, cardio then strength, for up to six days. Rest on Day Seven
Cardio and Strength on the same day	Do cardio and strength one day, rest the next and repeat for up to five days. Rest on Day Six and Day Seven

INTRODUCTION TO WORKOUTS

The next section is broken into three parts to correspond with the fitness tools - **Flexibility, Cardio and Strength**. Each one describes the benefits of the fitness tool and gives important information about it.

We have included **seven workouts** for you to try. Each workout has a different purpose - the first three are pure cardio workouts to exercise your heart and lungs while you torch calories. The third is for boosting your metabolism to aid with fat burning and increasing your stamina, strength and power. The fourth, fifth and sixth are for muscle building and toning. They will give you something to start with and help you get familiar with the gym and some of the equipment.

We have organized the workouts into an order of easiest to harder within the two sections - Cardio and Fat-burning, and Tone Up and Muscle Building - depending on what you want to focus on.

Please note, these are sample workouts. They are *NOT* personalized or tailor-made for you specifically, as that would take a professional trainer to test and measure your strengths and weaknesses, before prescribing what is best for you.

Before starting a new activity, including the workouts contained in this book, get a medical examination and read the information on the copyright page at the front of the book.

If you want a personalized or tailor-made program based on your strengths, weaknesses, health and fitness levels, please see your local certified and experienced personal trainer (see the chapter - *Choosing the Right Trainer* on page **32**)

STRETCHING AND FLEXIBILITY

FLEXIBILITY TRAINING
Good for Increasing Range of Motion

Stretching is the tool you use to increase range of motion (ROM) of muscles and around joints.

There are three reasons why people get tight, stiff or have a decrease in ROM in an area of the body:
- Muscles are kept in a shortened state over a long period of time (inactivity). An example is when you sit for long periods, the muscles in your lower back and the back of your legs (hamstrings) get tight
- Using muscles (being active). Any general use: walking, playing sports and so on can cause this
- Aging (you get the accumulation of 1 and 2 above), all the activity and inactivity of a lifetime add up to a natural decrease in joint fluidity and mobility

Whether you are active or inactive, it is a good idea to include stretching as part of your weekly activities. Stretching becomes more important especially as you age, and when you are very active.

Some benefits of stretching are:
- Increased flexibility
- Improved posture
- Preparation for vigorous activity
- Decreased chance of injury
- Recovery from injury

HOW TO STRETCH

Two of the most common ways to increase flexibility are dynamic and static stretching.

FLEXIBILITY TRAINING
Good for Increasing Range of Motion

DYNAMIC STRETCHING: Also known as movement stretching, is a type of stretching you do as part of your warm up before a workout or a sporting event. You stretch the specific muscles you are about to use in the sport, fitness class or during a strength workout.

Here's how you do dynamic stretching:

- Move the limb or torso through it's full *range of motion* (ROM) to a point of slight discomfort, without bouncing it at the end of the movement
- Repeat the movement 10 to 20 times, gradually increasing ROM and speed
- Stop when you no longer increase ROM.

Here's an example of how to use dynamic stretching for the back of the upper leg (hamstring).

- In a standing position swing one straight leg out in front of you several times (like a straight-legged soccer kick)
- Gradually increase the height of the leg
- Stop when it no longer increases in ROM

STATIC STRETCHING: Also known as hold stretching, is a common type of stretching that you do as part of your cool down after a workout or after participating in a sport. If you want to focus on static stretching as your workout, always make sure you are warmed up beforehand. Never stretch cold muscles.

FLEXIBILITY TRAINING
Good for Increasing Range of Motion

To do static stretching:

- Stretch the limb or torso slightly past its comfortable ROM without over-stretching
- Hold the muscle in the stretch position for 30 to 60 seconds When the muscles relax their tension and lengthen slightly, stretch further to a new point of slight discomfort. If the muscles don't relax their tension and lengthen, decrease the stretch a little until they do
- Repeat the stretch two more times, going a little further each time.

Here's an example of how to use static stretching for the back of the upper leg (hamstring).

- Stand on one leg and rest the other heel on a bench that is lower than your hips
- Bend forward from the hips and reach down your leg until you feel slight discomfort
- Hold the muscles in that stretch position for 30 to 60 seconds
- When the muscles relax their tension and lengthen slightly, stretch further to a new point of slight discomfort (if the muscles don't release their tension, decrease the stretch a little)
- Repeat two more times, each time stretching or going a little further

BASIC STRETCHES

You can use the following stretches as either static or dynamic stretches.

- Use **dynamic stretching at the start** of your workout, move gently in and out of each stretch (never bounce).
- Use **static stretching at the end** of your workout, hold each stretch for 30 to 60 seconds gradually increasing the stretch as you breathe.

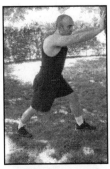
Calf stretch - push back heel down

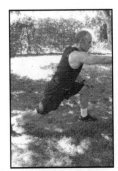
Front hip stretch - back heel up

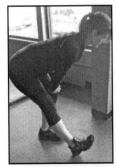
Hamstring stretch - back of leg

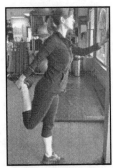
Quad stretch - front of thigh

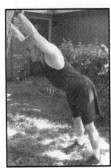
Shoulder/upper back stretch

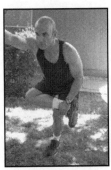
Glute and hip stretch

CARDIO AND FAT-BURNING WORKOUTS

51

CARDIO TRAINING
Good for the Heart, Good for Burning Calories

Cardio has many benefits, here are a few:

- Cardio helps prevent lots of diseases (diabetes, heart disease, high blood pressure, high cholesterol, to name a few)
- Cardio burns calories (running for ten minutes at six miles per hour burns about 100 calories)
- Cardio helps to reduce body fat
- Cardio helps the heart by increasing the size of the chambers and allowing it to pump more blood with each beat

HOW TO DO CARDIO WORKOUTS

Cardio exercise or activities are also known as aerobic exercise or sometimes endurance exercise. You will get cardio improvement if you do cardio exercise long or hard enough. There are several ways you can do cardio exercise:

GYM CARDIO MACHINES - You can do cardio at the gym on the treadmill, elliptical, bike, rower, hand crank, or stair master.

GROUP FITNESS CLASSES - Classes like the boxing class, dance fitness or circuit classes focus mostly on cardio exercise and can be a fun way to improve your cardio fitness.

BODY WEIGHT CARDIO - You can do a lot of body weight exercises (jogging on the spot with knees high every now and then, jogging heels up - butt kickers, "skating" side to side, burpees, mountain climbers and bear crawls) in short bursts of 30 to 60 seconds each to a total of three to ten minutes or more. This will create a cardio workout effect.

OUTDOOR CARDIO / SPORTS - Some outdoor cardio activities you can do are: walking fast, climbing stairs, jogging, swimming, hiking, cycling and rowing. Most sports, such as soccer, hockey, basketball, and some martial arts have a high ratio of cardio activity.

CARDIO TRAINING
Good for the Heart, Good for Burning Calories

There are two main ways to do cardio, this applies to indoor or outdoor cardio training.

STEADY STATE TRAINING - Also known as L.S.D. (long slow distance) training. This is what most people do for cardio. LSD cardio is where you work out at a certain speed, resistance, hill angle, number of strides or revolutions per minute for a given time.

INTERVAL TRAINING - Also known as hard to easy or high to low training. This is a less common type of cardio but gaining popularity as scientific research demonstrates its effectiveness in increasing cardio fitness levels fast. It is tougher, more challenging and a good change to regular LSD training.

If you are new to exercise, start with LSD training for 3-4 weeks then switch to some easier versions of interval training.

GET THE MOST OUT OF CARDIO TRAINING

It's important to vary your speed, resistance or level of difficulty, incline, and stride length when using the cardio machines. It's also important to switch up the type of cardio machine or bodyweight activity you choose to do.

Typical durations for a beginner or for someone who is quite unfit can be as little as two to five minutes at a time, building up to 30 minutes over several weeks.

CARDIO TRAINING
Good for the Heart, Good for Burning Calories

CARDIO AT THE GYM

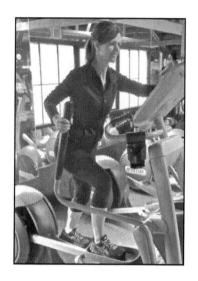

Elliptical training

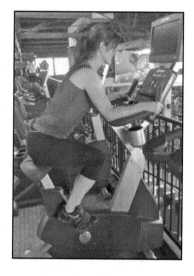

Stationary cycling

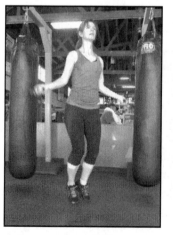

Jump rope

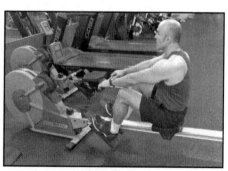

Rowing

CARDIO TRAINING
Good for the Heart, Good for Burning Calories

BEGINNER TREADMILL INTERVAL WORKOUT

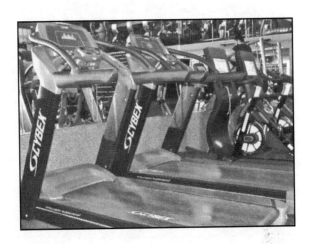

Warmup:
• 5 min walk (0 Incline) then 3 minute brisk walk (3 Incline)
Workout:
• *Hard Interval* - Very brisk walk at highest incline that can be sustained for 30 to 60 seconds
• *Easy Interval* - 60 to 90 seconds walk, easy pace at 0 Incline. Reduce the time to 30 seconds as you get fitter
• Start with 1 set of Hard/Easy and build up to 5 to 10 sets over 2 to 3 months.
Cool down:
• 5 min easy walk (0 Incline)

STEADY STATE CARDIO WORKOUT
Beginner to Intermediate Level

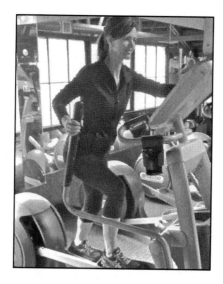

Here is a very simple cardio workout. To get best results, this would not be the only workout you'd do because it doesn't involve any strength development. You could **do it every second workout day** with good results. Cardio is great for helping to burn fat so it should be part of your overall workout plan if you are trying to lose weight.

Breathe - never hold your breath during any exercise.

1. **WARM-UP:** Pick a cardio machine and press the quick start button then the speed or level arrows to set it at a slow and relatively easy pace for about 5 minutes to warm up. You will go from the warmup right into the workout and *you will save your stretching until the end.*

STEADY STATE CARDIO WORKOUT

2. **WORKOUT:** Set the controls of your machine (using the up and down arrows) so you can continue using it for 30 to 50 minutes at a steady pace (you will be doing steady state cardio training). You want to be working at about 60 to 70% of your maximum effort, in other words, you want to be breathing fairly hard but never gasping for air or feeling dizzy or nauseous. If that happens, slow down until you recover.

(If you are new to exercise, start at 5 to 10 minutes and build up to 30 to 50 minutes over the next 1 to 3 months)

3. **STRETCH:** Do static/hold stretches. Stretch the whole body (see examples on page **49**)

Make sure you use different types of machines regularly when you do this kind of workout to avoid overuse injuries and to challenge different parts of your body. Use the treadmill one day, then the elliptical, then the stepper, for example. When you build up to doing more than 30 minutes at a time, you can also do 10 minutes on 3 different machines in one workout.

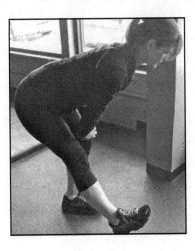

HIIT CARDIO WORKOUT
Intermediate to Advanced Level

After you have conquered the *Steady State Cardio Workout*, try the next level up - the *HIIT Cardio Workout*. Not only does it take less time, but it gets better results because it is more challenging. For this you will be doing **high intensity interval training** (HIIT) and you will be working quite a bit harder than when doing the *Steady State Cardio Workout*. To do this style of training, you should be relatively fit, so save it until you know your cardio fitness is up for it.

Breathe - never hold your breath during any exercise.

1. **WARM-UP:** Pick a cardio machine and, using the quick start button then the speed or level arrows, set it at a slow and relatively easy pace for about 5 minutes. You will go from the warmup right into the workout and *you will save your stretching until the end of the workout.*

2. **WORKOUT:**
   - *Hard interval* - go as fast and hard as you can at the highest resistance that can be sustained for 30 to 60 seconds (you will be working at 70 to 90% of maximal effort).
   - *Easy interval* - 30 to 60 seconds at the lowest resistance and a slow speed. This is when you recover your breathing and your heart rate slows.
   - You will continue doing these intervals for **10 to 15 minutes** then cool down with the machine set to the easy interval settings for 5 minutes.

3. **STRETCH:** Do static/hold stretches. Stretch the whole body (see examples on page **49**)

TOTAL BODY METABOLIC WORKOUT
Intermediate to Advanced Level

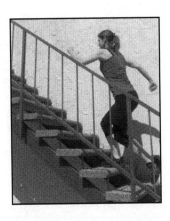

This workout is designed to help you improve your cardio fitness and strength while simultaneously torching calories for effective fat loss. If you are new to working out, start easy and move slowly and if you experience joint or nerve pain, stop.

Breathe - never hold your breath during any exercise.

1. **WARM-UP:** Do ten minutes of cardio. Use the treadmill, elliptical or bike. You want to reach a state of breathing hard but still being able to talk. You should notice your heart rate increasing and you should break into a light sweat.

2. **STRETCH:** Do gentle movement-type stretches (see examples on page **49**).

3. **WORKOUT:** After you do the first exercise, move on to the next one and so on, in a circuit. Give yourself 30 to 60 seconds between exercises. Start with one round of the whole circuit and build up to three or four rounds as you get fitter and stronger.

There are exercise descriptions and pictures on the following pages to make it easier for you to do the workout.

TOTAL BODY METABOLIC WORKOUT

Exercise #1: Burpees

From standing position, squat down and walk or jump your feet back until you are in a plank position, then walk or jump your feet forward to start position. Stand up and repeat. **Do 10 to 20 repetitions.**

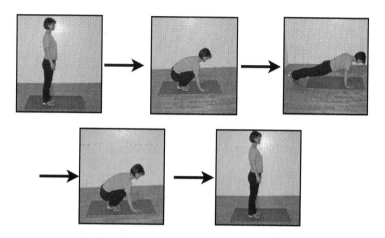

Exercise #2: Push-ups

Beginners do standing push-ups off a wall, otherwise do push-ups from your knees or toes. Never let your midsection sag, keep your shoulders over your hands and make sure your head doesn't drop. **Do 10 to 20 repetitions.**

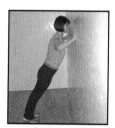 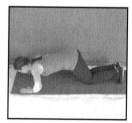 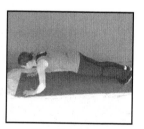

Standing Push-up   Knee Push-up   Toe Push-up

TOTAL BODY METABOLIC WORKOUT

Exercise #3: Side Shuffles
Move quickly sideways - 10 steps to the right then 10 steps to the left. Keep your knees bent.
Do for 30 to 60 seconds.

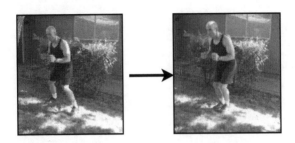

Exercise #4: Squats
Keep feet pointed straight ahead, hip-width apart. Maintain the natural curve of the lower back and neck. Squat until the angle at your knees is about 90 degrees. Never lock your knee joints or hold your breath.
Do 10 to 20 repetitions.

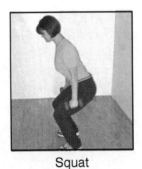
Squat

TOTAL BODY METABOLIC WORKOUT

Exercise #5: Bear Crawls

Start face down with your hands and feet on the ground and "walk" forwards like a bear for 6 steps then "walk" backwards in the same way. You can vary this by "walking" sideways as well.

Breathe - don't hold your breath.

Do for 30 to 60 seconds.

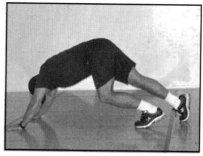

Bear Crawl

4. **COOL-DOWN:** Use one of the cardio machines for 3 to 10 minutes, taking it easy to bring your heart rate back down.

5. **STRETCH:** Do static/hold stretches. Stretch the whole body (see examples on page **49**)

TONING, SCULPTING, STRENGTH
AND MUSCLE-BUILDING WORKOUTS

STRENGTH TRAINING
Good For Strength, Toning and Muscle Building

Strength training (also known as weight training and resistance training) is what you do to build and maintain muscle tissue in your body.

Strength training and strength exercises can be a lot of fun to do. There are many benefits to strength training, from looking and feeling better, to functioning better in everything you do.

AGING AND LOSS OF FUNCTION

As your body ages it gradually loses a very important commodity: muscle tissue. If you lose too much muscle, your body dies in quality and in actuality - simple tasks like walking up steps or climbing into bed can become very difficult and painful, your balance is badly affected so falling can become a problem. People who lack muscle tissue look saggy and soft, it's muscle that gives you a toned and healthy look and it's muscle that gives your body a pleasing shape (whether you are a man or a woman). Strength training, also known as weight training and resistance training, is what you do to maintain and build muscle tissue to keep your body healthy, strong and looking great.

Some benefits of strength training are:
• Looking good
• Increased physical strength so you can do more physically in your life
• Toned muscles
• Improved physical shape and appearance
• Increased fat loss potential - muscle cells use more calories than fat cells
• Faster metabolism - you burn more energy all day, every day

STRENGTH TRAINING
Good For Strength, Toning and Muscle Building

There are 3 basic ways you can do strength training and with each type you can progress from very easy to very difficult exercises.

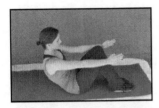

BODY WEIGHT STRENGTH TRAINING - Sit ups, push-ups, chin ups, squats, and dips, for example

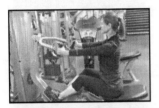

MACHINES - Seated row, leg press, chest press, and lat pulldown, for example

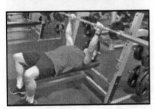

FREE WEIGHTS - Bench press, barbell squats, and barbell dead-lifts, for example

A simple way to start strength training is by doing body weight exercises, then include some machine exercises. As you increase your core and limb strength, you can go on to the more advanced free weights exercises. Using free weights takes more skill, balance and strength than using machines or your own body weight.

STRENGTH TRAINING
BODY WEIGHT

The beauty of body weight strength training is that it can be done anywhere, including the gym. All you need is some space, your body and an understanding of how to do the the exercises.

Of course, knowing the correct form for body weight exercises is very important. So is knowing how to make them easier to do (for when you are beginning) and how to make them more difficult (as your strength increases).

BODY WEIGHT CORE EXERCISES

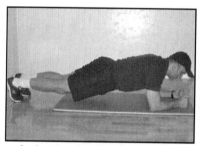

A simple plank - this exercise targets the core

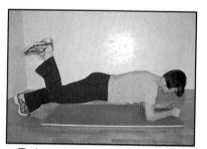

To increase the difficulty, lift a foot off the ground

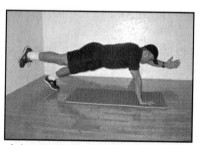

Advanced plank - one hand and one foot off the floor

BODY WEIGHT 101 WORKOUT
Beginner to Intermediate Level

This is a total body strength workout. It's what we like to call the "low tech, high return on your investment" workout. It can be done anywhere, anytime and if it's done right, can yield excellent results.

Breathe - never hold your breath during any exercise.

1. **WARM-UP:** Do ten minutes of cardio. Jog on the spot, do jumping jacks or stair runs. You want to reach a state of breathing hard but still being able to talk. You should notice your heart rate increasing and you should break into a light sweat.

2. **STRETCH:** Do gentle movement-type stretches (see examples on page **49**).

3. **WORKOUT:** Beginners start with 5 reps (repetitions) and gradually build up to 20 reps of each exercise. Add rest between as needed. Do 1 set (round or circuit) and build up to 2 or 3 sets. For those who want to add a cardio element and are more advanced, add 30 to 60 seconds of jogging, jump rope, hopping, mountain climbers, or burpees in between sets.

Exercise #1: Squats

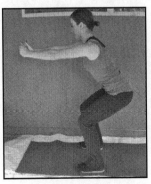

Place your feet about hip width apart and, with your knees staying in line with your feet (not caving in), take your hips back as you bend your knees. Make sure to keep your abdominals braced and strong. Hands can be by your sides, above your head or held in front of you at shoulder height.

BODY WEIGHT 101 WORKOUT
Beginner to Intermediate Level

Exercise #2: Push-ups

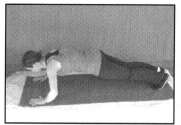

Place hands slightly wider than shoulder width apart. Lower chest to about 1 inch off the ground then press up. Keep abdominals braced and strong. Do push-ups off a wall or bench until you can do floor push-ups

Exercise # 3: Hanging Pull-ups

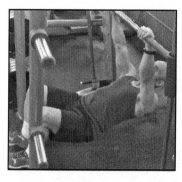

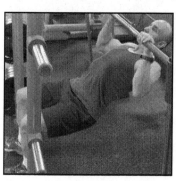

Set the bar between waist to chest height then place your hands shoulder-width apart with an overhand grip on the bar. Lower your body so the bar is in line with your shoulders and your feet are on the ground hip-width apart. The further out your feet are, the more difficult this exercise becomes. When you pull up, keep your abs engaged, chest out and shoulders back.

BODY WEIGHT 101 WORKOUT
Beginner to Intermediate Level

Exercise # 4: Criss-cross

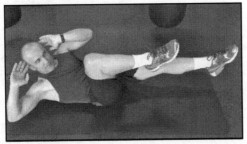

Lying face up, hands by ears, elbows out. Crunch up, twist and bring an elbow to the opposite knee. Switch elbow and knee and repeat.

Exercise # 5: Superman

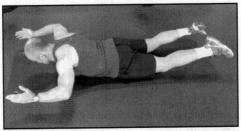

Lying face down, lift your chest and legs off the ground and hold for a couple of seconds then lower to the ground again. Try to keep your neck in a neutral position.

4. **COOL-DOWN:** Use one of the cardio machines for 3 to 10 minutes, taking it easy to bring your heart rate back down.

5. **STRETCH:** Do static/hold stretches. Stretch the whole body (see examples on page **49**)

STRENGTH TRAINING
MACHINES

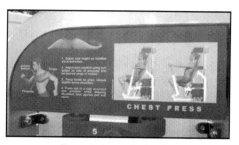

1. Read the instructions

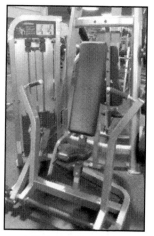

2. Look for all
adjustments

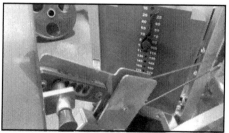

3. Make all adjustments and
choose the weight

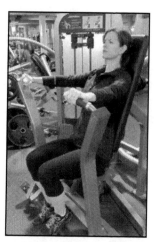

4. Do the exercise

STRENGTH TRAINING
MACHINES

- Locate the instruction diagram on the machine you want to learn to use (most modern machines have an instruction diagram. Beware, not all are 100% correct)

- Look at the muscles that are colored in the diagram, indicating the muscles the machine is targeting

- Read the instructions on how to set up or use the machine

- Stand back from the machine and look for all possible adjustments that can be made to customize the machine to suit your body (adjustments may be for seat height, depth, handle width, handle depth, etc)

- Make all the the necessary adjustments to customize the machine as much as possible for your physical size and body type so that your body is placed correctly, like the diagram shows

- Choose a weight for the exercise so that you can do 10 to 20 repetitions (or movements) without over-exerting yourself. Start at 50 to 70% of your maximal effort if you are new, injury free and have medical clearance to exercise

- Wipe the machine down before and after you use it and use a towel to sit or lie down on the machine

- Do the exercise on the machine with a slow and deliberate cadence. For example, **work at a tempo of 2:2:2 seconds meaning 2 seconds down, hold 2 seconds, and up 2 seconds.** This equals one repetition (rep)

- Breathe gently throughout the rep

- If you feel pain, stop and get professional help

MACHINE WEIGHTS 101 WORKOUT
Beginner to Intermediate Level

This is a simple machine strength workout. It is designed to increase muscle mass and works your entire body. Here are some reasons why you should want to increase your muscle mass with strength training:

- Look good - nothing better than a well-shaped body
- Increase physical strength so you can do more in your life
- Tone your body - tighten those flabby bits
- Improve your physical shape and appearance
- Increase your fat loss potential - muscle tissue uses more calories than other tissues in the body
- Speed up your metabolism - your whole body works better when its muscles are challenged with strength training

Breathe - never hold your breath during any exercise.

1. **WARM-UP:** Do ten minutes of cardio. Use the treadmill, elliptical or bike. You want to reach a state of breathing hard but still being able to talk. You should notice your heart rate increasing and you should break into a light sweat.

2. **STRETCH:** Do gentle movement-type stretches (see examples on page **49**).

3. **WORKOUT:** Do 2 to 3 sets of each exercise with a 1 minute rest between sets, then move onto the next exercise. You can also add burpees or bear crawls between sets to help burn more calories and speed your metabolism.

Note on breathing: Do not hold your breath for any length of time doing strength exercises. Breathe out during exertion or the toughest part of the exercise.

MACHINE WEIGHTS 101 WORKOUT

Exercise #1: Leg Press

This exercise works your thighs, calves and butt. It's a good lower body exercise that keeps your spine in a safe position. Make sure you adjust the leg press settings so the machine fits your body. *Start with a low weight* and do 10 to 20 repetitions. If that was very easy, increase the weight gradually until you find a weight you can do that's challenging - you want it to be about 70% of your maximal effort.

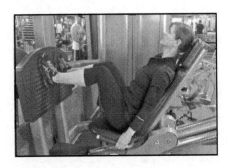

Exercise #2: Chest Press

This exercise works the chest muscles as well as the arms and shoulders. Make sure you adjust the chest press machine settings so it fits your body. *Start with a low weight* and do 10 to 20 repetitions. If that was very easy, increase the weight gradually until you find a weight you can do that's challenging - you want it to be about 70% of your maximal effort.

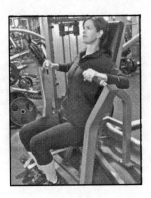

MACHINE WEIGHTS 101 WORKOUT

Exercise #3: Seated Row

This exercise works the upper back and arms. You will also work the abdominal muscles when you use correct form. Make sure you adjust the settings of the seated row machine so it fits your body. *Start with a low weight* and do 10 to 20 repetitions. If that was very easy, increase the weight gradually until you find a weight you can do that's challenging - you want it to be about 70% of your maximal effort.

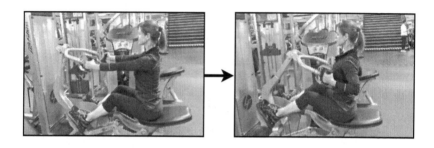

Exercise #4: Abdominals Machine

This exercise works the abdominal muscles. Lie on the bench with your feet up and elbows resting on the bars. *Start with your torso lower on the bench* and do 10 to 20 repetitions. If that was very easy, move your torso up the bench until you find a position that's challenging - you want it to be about 70% of your maximal effort.

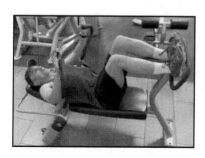
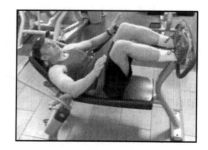

MACHINE WEIGHTS 101 WORKOUT

Exercise #5: Lower Back Machine
This exercise works the lower back as well as glutes and
hamstrings. Make sure you adjust the settings of the lower
back machine so it fits your body. *Start with your arms close
to your body* and do 10 to 20 repetitions. If that was very easy,
increase change your arm position until you find a position you
can do that's challenging - you want it to be about 70% of your
maximal effort. Try hands by ears, elbows wide (as shown) or
arms straight and in line with your ears.

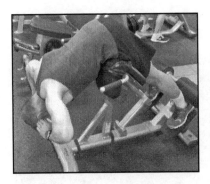 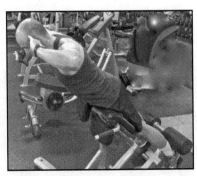

4. **COOL-DOWN:** Use one of the cardio machines for 3 to 10
   minutes, taking it easy to bring your heart rate back down.

5. **STRETCH:** Do static/hold stretches. Stretch the whole
   body (see examples on page **49**)

STRENGTH TRAINING
FREE WEIGHTS

Free weights are more advanced than machine or most
bodyweight exercises so it's a good idea to hire an experienced
and competent certified trainer to teach you the correct way to
use free weights. This way you can get the most out of the free
weights and maximize safety to avoid injury.

Always use excellent exercise form (this goes for all exercises,
but is even more important when using free weights). A good
starting tempo is 2:2:2 (2 seconds down, 2 seconds hold, 2
seconds up). Use safety clips on the ends of the bar bell to
make sure the plates don't accidentally fall off and hurt you.

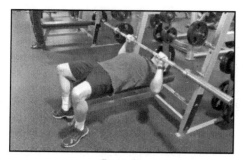

Bar bell

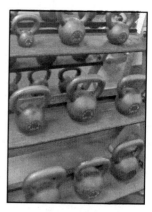

Kettle bells

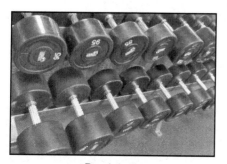

Dumb bells

FREE WEIGHTS 101 WORKOUT
Intermediate to Advanced Level

Here is a good, simple free weights workout aimed at building muscle and working out your entire body. Free weights take more skill than machines because you have to control the weights yourself, you don't get help from cables to keep the weights in the correct place as they move.

Always start with a light weight when learning a free weights exercise. Performing the exercise with correct form is essential to make sure you get the full benefit of the exercise and you don't get injured.

Investing in some sessions with a competent personal trainer is a very good idea to make sure you are using free weights correctly.

1. **WARM-UP:** Do ten minutes of cardio. Use the treadmill, elliptical, bike or do bodyweight exercises. You want to reach a state of breathing hard but still being able to talk. You should notice your heart rate increasing and you should break into a light sweat.

2. **STRETCH:** Do gentle movement-type stretches (see examples on page **49**).

3. **WORKOUT:** Do 2 to 3 sets of 10 to 20 repetitions of each exercise with a 1 minute rest between sets, then move onto the next exercise. Add burpees, bear crawls or jogging on the spot between sets to help burn fat and speed your metabolism.

Intensity - 50% to 70% to start then build up to 80% to 90% over the next three months.

Note on breathing: Do not hold your breath for any length of time doing strength exercises. Breathe out during exertion or the toughest part of the exercise.

FREE WEIGHTS 101 WORKOUT

Exercise #1: Barbell Bench Press

Lie face-up on the bench with feet on ground for stability. Use an overhand grip with hands placed slightly wider than shoulders (see picture). Lower the bar slowly to about 1 inch from your chest then push it back to the start position. Never lock your elbows. Try to keep your back on the bench. *Start with a low weight* and do 10 to 20 repetitions. If that was very easy, increase the weight gradually until you find a weight you can do that's challenging - you want it to be about 50 to 70% of your maximal effort to start off with.

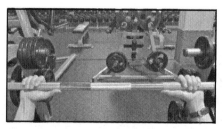

Hand position

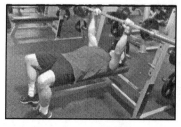 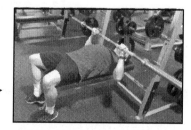

Start: extend arms but don't
lock your elbows

Slowly lower bar to 1 inch off
chest

The bench press works your chest muscles, the front of your shoulders and triceps.

FREE WEIGHTS 101 WORKOUT

Exercise #2: Barbell Bent Over Row

Stand with legs slightly bent and feet hip width apart and parallel. Hold the bar with your palms facing back and slightly wider than shoulder width. Keeping your back in a neutral position (natural curves), lean forward until the bar is about knee level (this is your start position) then, bending your elbows, "row" the bar so it comes close to your navel then slowly return to the start position. *Start with a low weight* and do 10 to 20 repetitions. If that was very easy, increase the weight gradually until you find a weight you can do that's challenging - you want it to be about 70% of your maximal effort.

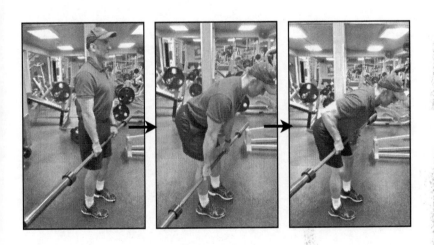

The bent over row works a lot of back muscles, including the trapezius, back of the shoulders and lats. It also works the abs, and biceps.

FREE WEIGHTS 101 WORKOUT

Exercise #3: Barbell Squat

With your feet hip-width apart, stand under the barbell while it is on the rack. Rest the bar across the back of your shoulders (not the neck), it should be on soft tissue, not bone. Place your hands on the bar. Step back a few steps with the bar, place your feet about hip-width apart and slowly squat making sure your spine maintains its neutral curve (no hunching). Engage your butt muscles and abs. When your thighs are about 90 degrees at the knee, straighten your legs and return to standing position. *Start with a low weight* and do 10 to 20 repetitions. If that was very easy, increase the weight gradually until you find a weight you can do that's challenging - you want it to be about 70% of your maximal effort.

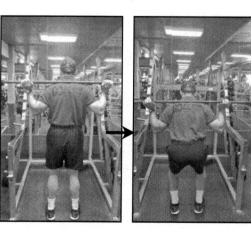 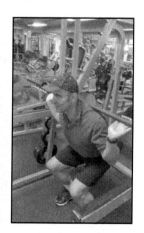

The squat is known as the "king of exercises" because it uses nearly all the muscles of the body as well as the heart and lungs. It is especially good for working the butt muscles (glutes), legs, abs and back muscles.

FREE WEIGHTS 101 WORKOUT

Exercise # 4: Dumbbell Curls

Stand with your feet hip-width apart, a slight bend in your knees. Hold the dumbbells with palms facing forward and arms extended. Bend the elbows to raise the forearms, try to keep your elbows still and close to your sides. Slowly bring your hands back to the start position and repeat. *Start with a low weight* and do 10 to 20 repetitions. If that was very easy, increase the weight gradually until you find a weight you can do that's challenging - you want it to be about 70% of your maximal effort.

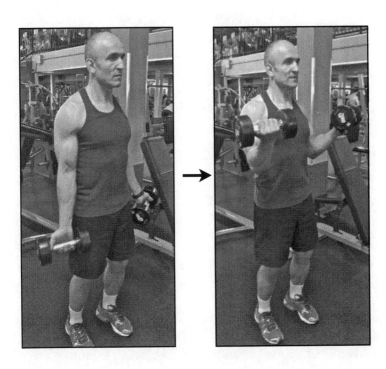

FREE WEIGHTS 101 WORKOUT

Exercise # 5: Bench Dips

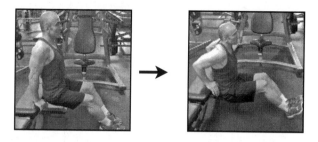

Place your hands on either side of your hips on the bench.
Your hips should be just off the edge of the bench. Slowly lower
your hips until your elbows are about 90 degrees then press up
until your arms are almost straight - don't lock out your
elbows. Try to keep your hips close to the bench throughout
the movement.

Exercise # 6: Dumbbell Shoulder Press

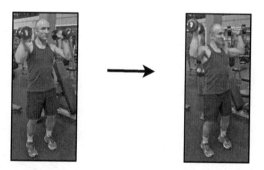

Stand with feet hip width apart and a slight bend at the knees.
Hold dumbbells in a hammer grip at shoulder height. Press up
until dumbbells are at head height then bring them back to the
starting position.

Doing presses in this way, instead of fully extending the arms
above the head, isolates the shoulder muscles and helps
prevent injury.

FREE WEIGHTS 101 WORKOUT

4. **COOL-DOWN:** Use one of the cardio machines for 3 to 10 minutes, taking it easy to bring your heart rate back down.

5. **STRETCH:** Do static/hold stretches. Stretch the whole body (see examples on page **49**)

AVOIDING PLATEAUS AND BOREDOM

You should change up your workouts every six to eight weeks to avoid plateaus, boredom and lack of results.

The body responds best when it's challenged and given different things to do. Doing the exact same thing for months or even years results in a plateau - no progress. You can avoid a plateau and the risk of getting bored and not getting results by changing your workout program.

If you change your workout routine every time you go to the gym, you will not get very strong in any one exercise.

Getting good coaching is a smart way to make sure you are doing exercises properly - on one hand you want to keep things safe and on the other hand you want to get the most out of every movement you make.

PART FIVE - DIET

IMPROVE YOUR DIET

Here's a simple diagram to show you how to eat throughout the day so you can maintain your energy levels and avoid putting on unwanted weight.

The Eat Smart Pyramid (ESP)

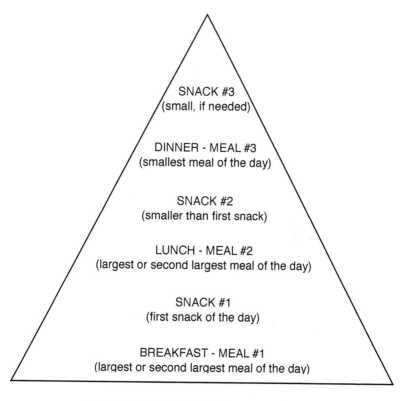

SNACK #3
(small, if needed)

DINNER - MEAL #3
(smallest meal of the day)

SNACK #2
(smaller than first snack)

LUNCH - MEAL #2
(largest or second largest meal of the day)

SNACK #1
(first snack of the day)

BREAKFAST - MEAL #1
(largest or second largest meal of the day)

**START AT THE BOTTOM OF THE PYRAMID
AND WORK YOUR WAY UP**

All meals and snacks should include all three
nutrients: protein, carbohydrate and fats

IMPROVE YOUR DIET
EAT RIGHT TO CHANGE YOUR BODY

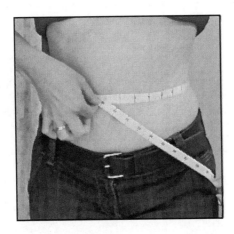

For Weight Loss - Fat Loss:
- Eat a little less than usual each day (250 to 500 calories)
- Cut sugar out of your diet
- Cut starchy, processed foods like white bread and pasta out of your diet
- Eat lean proteins, lots of leafy green vegetables, healthy fats
- Do daily cardio and strength training
- Make sure you drink 8 to 12 glasses of water daily

For Building Muscle:
- Eat 250 to 500 calories more than usual
- Eat 1 to 1.5 grams of protein per kilogram of body weight
- Eat plenty of vegetables and some fats
- Do basic strength training - squats, dead lifts and bench press are excellent for building total body muscle
- Take basic supplements - whey protein, creatine, L-glutamine, branch chain amino acids (BCAAs)

IMPROVE YOUR DIET
EAT RIGHT TO CHANGE YOUR BODY

Here are some examples of healthy protein, fat and carbohydrates to eat no matter whether you want to build muscle or lose weight.

PROTEIN	FAT	CARBOHYDRATE
eggs	nuts nut butters	salads and vegetables
fish	avocado	sweet potato
chicken	olive oil	quinoa
protein powder	coconut oil	oats
steak	cheeses	fruit

Not everybody eats the same way. Depending on your age, genetics, general health or metabolism, your diet can be the most important factor in helping you achieve your goals. Be willing to make changes and improvements to the way you eat.

There is a lot of information on food and diet in other books. We are providing a very short summary in this book, to point you in the right direction.

INDEX

A

aerobic, 8, 18, 52

B

baby boomers, 3, 20
body weight exercises, 7, 52, 65, 66
bodybuilding, viii, 16, 17

C

cardio, 1, 6, 8, 20, 11-13, 15, 23, 28, 34-36, 39, 41-43, 51-59, 62, 67, 69, 72, 75, 77, 83, 87
clothing, 23, 24, 26
cool down, 24, 26, 34, 35, 39, 47, 55, 58

D

diet, 1, 13, 20, 22, 23, 85-88
disease, 10, 14, 28, 52

E

energy, xi, xii, 8, 10, 12, 20, 64, 86
etiquette, 21, 27-29
exercise, ii, iii, ix, x, xi, xii, 3, 7-11, 14-16, 20, 22-24, 28, 29, 31-34, 36-39, 42, 43, 52, 53, 56-62, 64-83

F

fat-burning, 41, 43, 51
fitness, iii, v, vi, ix-xii, 1-3, 6-12, 20, 26, 32, 33, 42, 43, 47, 52, 53, 58, 59
flexibility, 6, 9, 11, 35, 41, 42, 45, 46, 47, 48
free weights, 7, 63, 65, 76-83
four steps to success, 14, 17

G

goals, x, 1-6, 11, 12, 20, 22, 26, 33, 37, 42
gym, viii, ix, xi, xii, 1, 2, 4, 5, 8, 13, 16-18, 21-29, 33, 41-43, 52, 54, 66, 83
gym membership, 1, 2, 42

INDEX

WE WOULD LOVE TO HEAR FROM YOU

Thank you for buying our book. We're sure that if you read it through and follow the instructions, you will have a good idea of what to do in the gym, know how to get along with other gym members and where to go for more help if you need it.

Would you mind taking a few minutes to write something on Amazon about this book? We check all our reviews and value the feedback, it helps us so much if we know what you got out of what we've put together for you.

Just type the name of this book in the Amazon search bar and scroll down to "write customer review".

You can always contact us. Our website is **www.gofitnow.com** and if you want to write, you can email us at **rudi@gofitnow.com**.

We'd love to hear what you liked most in the book, if there's anything you'd like added in the next edition, and how you're doing at the gym.

Thanks so much and the best of gym success to you!

Rudi and Tracey

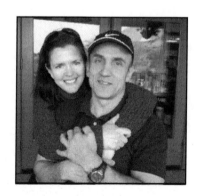

IF YOU LIKED THIS BOOK, YOU MIGHT ALSO ENJOY

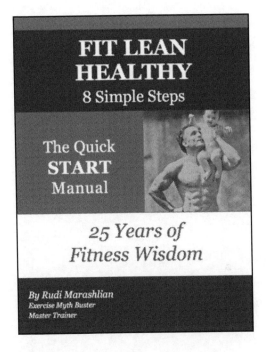

Fit Lean Healthy, 8 Simple Steps

- Discover your personal reasons and motivations for getting into shape
- Learn which activities you should be doing to achieve your specific personal fitness goals
- Work out what's stopping you - it's not the same for everyone
- Get a complete understanding of what food does to your body and how you should be eating to transform your body for good
- Learn how to test your strength, flexibility and overall fitness as well as your fat to lean ratio (much healthier than relying on the scales)

Visit **www.fitleanhealthy.com** to get this book.

Made in the USA
San Bernardino, CA
20 November 2017